Bibliographic information published by the German National Library:

The German National Library lists this publication in the National Bibliography; detailed bibliographic data are available on the Internet at http://dnb.dnb.de .

Imprint:

Print and binding: Books on Demand GmbH, Norderstedt Germany
ISBN: 978-3-668-02419-9

This book at GRIN:

http://www.grin.com/en/e-book/303837/implementation-of-an-evidence-based-practice-to-prevent-pressure-ulcers

Antje Dangel

Implementation of an Evidence-Based Practice to Prevent Pressure Ulcers

GRIN Publishing

Implementation of a Practice Change:

An Evidence-Based Practice Project to Prevent Pressure Ulcers

Antje Dangel

University of South Florida

Table of Contents

Introduction

Pressure ulcers, caused by prolonged immobility, are increasing among hospital patients. They can cause patient discomfort and infection, may increase treatment time, length of hospital admission, medical bills, and can potentially cause death (AHRQ, 2009). Current guidelines recommended by the AHRQ aid nursing staff in pressure ulcer prevention; however, the combination of specialty skin products, silicone dressings, and a 4-hour turning schedule may prevent pressure ulcers entirely.

PICOT Question

To identify a need for change, and to develop a change in practice project, the following PICOT question was developed. In the adult cardiac patient population, how does the preventative use of natural cleansers and nutrient emollients, the application of foam dressings, and a 4-hour turning schedule in comparison to the use of aloe vesta soap and lotion alone, no dressings, and a 2- or 3-hour turning schedule affect the rate of pressure ulcer development within three months?

Infrastructure to Support Change

Sarasota Memorial Healthcare System, a magnet recognized not-for-profit organization, is committed to delivering safe, high-quality care that results in desired outcomes and is consistent with current professional knowledge (Mission Statement/Vision, para. 4). The organizational culture is reflected in the mission statement as well as the organization's participation with several agencies including The Joint Commission, the Agency for Healthcare Research and Quality Patient Safety Indicators, the American Nurses Credentialing Center Magnet Program (Sarasota Memorial Quality Report, para.4), and many other health care accrediting agencies. Interdisciplinary collaboration is encouraged as evidenced by interdisciplinary meetings that focus on identifying the need for change and implementing evidence-based practice (EBP). Change that results in improved patient outcomes is encouraged by the executive team, risk management, nurse educators, several practice councils, and unit managers. Initiation of and participation in change is recognized by "nurse of clinical excellence" awards. At SMH, proposed changes are commonly presented to unit practice councils (UPC) throughout the organization. Council members vote on the proposed change, and if the majority of the UPC members and council chair agree upon the proposal, the specified change in practice is implemented systematically.

Summary of Synthesized Literature Review of Current Recommended Practice

Literature Search

PubMed, NCBI, and CINHAL were used to find research containing relevant information and clinical guidelines regarding pressure ulcer prevention. The key terms used in this search were *pressure ulcer*, *prevention*, *border foam dressing*, and *critical patient*.

Three peer-reviewed articles and one clinical guideline were selected for evaluation and synthesis.

Synthesis

Examination of the literature discussing pressure ulcer prevention has demonstrated that rates of pressure ulcer development can be reduced. Bergstrom et al. (2013) found that a 4-hour turning schedule is sufficient in pressure ulcer prevention. Santamaria et al. (2013) found that the application of soft silicone multi-layered foam dressings led to a 10% reduction rate of pressure ulcer development. Shannon et al. (2012) found that the use of a Pressure Ulcer Prevention

Program (PUPP) led to a 67% incidence reduction as it pertains to pressure ulcer development in nursing homes.

Proposed Practice Change

Collectively, the literature recommends utilization of specialty skin care products, silicone adhesive dressings, and a 4-hour turning schedule in order to prevent pressure ulcers. This intervention should be implemented in conjunction with current clinical guidelines recommended by the AHRQ. Cardio-vascular progressive care units (CVPCUs) should continue to conduct quarterly prevalence studies to record demographic and clinical data pertaining to pressure ulcer rates.

Change Strategy

Promoting Engagement

Nurses, nursing aids, unit managers, clinical coordinators, and physicians should participate in the change process. Kotter and Cohen's organizational change model should be utilized. Unit managers need to identify innovators, and individuals who have shown to be early adapters in the past to create a sense of urgency and promote and guide change (Melnyk & Fineout-Overholt, 2011). Stakeholders should communicate the vision and change strategy openly and individuals need to be empowered to express concerns and skepticism. Once barriers are recognized, stakeholders can develop a strategic plan, provide staff with evidence and start implementing change (Melnyk & Fineout-Overholt, 2011).

The Model for Evidence-Based Practice Change

Once stakeholders create a sense of urgency and establish uniform guidelines based on current evidence, EBP can be implemented into the clinical setting. SMH's stakeholders adhere to Kotter and Cohen's Model of Change (Melnyk & Fineout-Overholt, 2011) to implement change.

Roll Out Plan

Steps	Definition	Timeframe for Rollout
Step 1	Assess the need for practice change - Include stakeholders - Collect internal data about current practice - Compare external with internal data - Identify the problem - Link problem, interventions, and outcomes	Completed January, 2014
Step 2	Locate the best evidence - Identify types and sources - Review research concepts - Plan the search - Conduct the search	Completed February, 2014
Step 3	Critically analyze the evidence - Appraise and weigh the evidence - Synthesize the best evidence - Assess feasibility, benefits, and risks of new practice	Completed March, 2014
Step 4	Design of practice change - Define proposed change - Identify needed resources - Design the evaluation of the pilot - Design the implementation plan	Completed March, 2014
Step 5	Implement and evaluate change in practice - Implement pilot study - Evaluate processes, outcomes, and costs - Develop conclusions and recommendations	Implement May, 2014 Evaluate August, 2014
Step 6	Integrate and maintain change in practice - Communicate recommended change to stakeholders - Integrate into standards of practice - Monitor process and outcomes periodically - Celebrate and disseminate results of project	August, 2014

Project Evaluation

Beginning in May, all patients who undergo open-heart surgery will follow guidelines that include the applications of specialty skin products, silicone adhesive border dressings, and a 4-hour turning schedule to prevent the development of pressure ulcers. Designated staff will collect data via quarterly prevalence studies on all patients who undergo open-heart surgery. The project evaluation will be made by comparing the quarterly rate of pressure ulcer development before and after the initiation of the practice change.

Dissemination of EBP

Dissemination of this practice change can occur in several ways. First, written communication via email should happen with the executive team, the EBP council members and unit managers. SMH uses online learning modules when topics need to be introduced or refreshed. The new pressure ulcer prevention strategy can be conveyed through these online learning modules and PowerPoint presentations. Subsequently, service specific policies should and will be updated and conveyed during practice council meetings. Melnyk & Fineout-Overholt (2011) recommend the development of a journal club; clinical educators should be involved to nurture a positive learning environment. PowerPoint presentations as well as online learning modules can aid in transferring knowledge to adjunct facilities.

Methods of deliberate communication to other facilities regarding practice change may include visuals such as diagrams displaying before and after prevalence study results. This marketing strategy could be used during UPC meetings, and should include direct recognition of employees who champion the change. Information sharing outside SMH may include discussion or presentations at partnership meetings hosted by the Suncoast Organization of Nurse Executives (SCONE). As a major health care stakeholder, SMH's manager of the cardio-vascular step-down unit attends SCONE meetings on a quarterly basis. SMH also frequently communicates via email with other partners and Magnet facilities where change in practice and performance improvement is championed.

References

Agency for Healthcare Research and Quality. (2009). *Pressure ulcers are increasing among hospital patients: Research Activities.* Retrieved from http://archive.ahrq.gov/news/newsletters/research-activities/jan09/0109RA22.html

Bergstrom, N., Horn, S. D., Rapp, M., Stern, A., Barrett, R., & Watkiss, M. (2013). Turning for ulcer reduction: A multisite randomized clinical trial in nursing homes. *Journal of the American Geriatrics Society, 61*(10), 1705-1713. doi:10.1111/jgs.12440

Melnyk, B. M., & Fineout-Overholt, E. (2011). *Evidence-Based Practice in Nursing & Healthcare* (2nd ed.). Philadelphia, PA: Wolters Kluwer Lippincott Williams & Williams.

Santamaria, N., Gerdtz, M., Sage, S., McCann, J., Freeman, A., Vassiliou, T., … Knott, J. (27 May 2013). A randomized controlled trial of the effectiveness of soft silicone multi-layered foam dressings in the prevention of sacral and heel pressure ulcers in trauma and critically ill patients: The border trial. *International Wound Journal.* doi: 10.1111/iwj.12101

Sarasota Memorial Hospital. (2014). *Mission Statement / Vision.* Retrieved from http://smh.com/p.aspx?p=2

Sarasota Memorial Hospital. (2014). *Sarasota Memorial Quality Report.* Retrieved from http://www.smh.com/p.aspx?p=248

Shannon, R., Brown, L., & Chakravarthy, D. (2012). Pressure ulcer prevention program study: A randomized, controlled prospective comparative value evaluation of 2 pressure ulcer prevention strategies in nursing and rehabilitation centers. *Advances in Skin & Wound Care, 25*(10), 450-464.